STRONGFORT - INTELLIGENCE IN PHYSICAL CULTURE

(Original Version, Restored)

by

MAX UNGER

Originally Published in 1910

PUBLISHED BY O'Faolain Patriot L L C, Copyright 2012

info@physicalculturebooks.com

ISBN-13: 9781475016048

ISBN-10:1475016042

Published in the United States of America

To Order More Copies Visit:
PhysicalCultureBooks.com

appropriate for the reader's needs or expectations. The publisher expressly disclaims any and all responsibility and/or liabilities that might result from the uninformed or misinformed application of the techniques identified herein as well as for any unsupervised physical fitness training.

Finally, the publisher disclaims any and all liabilities arising from the use of any equipment featured in this book and makes no representations as to the utility, safety, or adequacy of the equipment generally or with respect to any specific purpose.

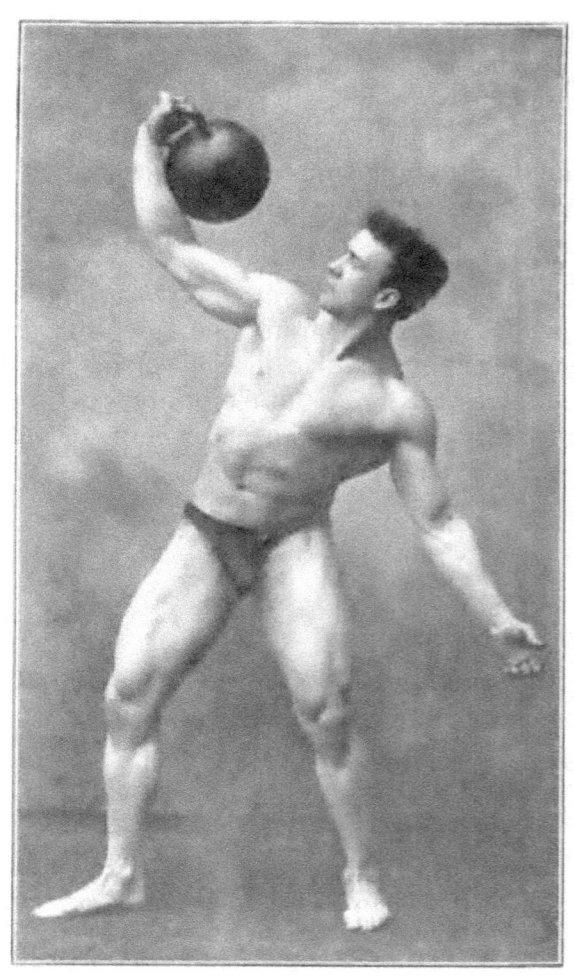

MAX UNGER

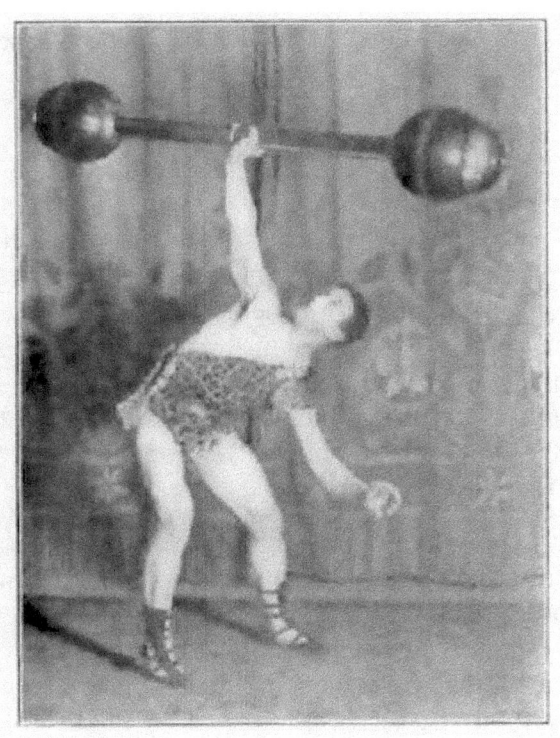

MAX UNGER LIFTING OVER HEAD A BAR-BELL
WEIGHING 312 POUNDS, THE WORLD'S RECORD.

FOREWORD BY CARL EASTON WILLIAMS

Formerly Associate Editor of Physical Culture
Magazine

Mr. Max Unger, better known throughout European countries as "Lionel Strongfort", is, so far as can be ascertained, the strongest man of all modern times. What the strength of some of the ancients may have been is difficult to determine definitely, though it is unlikely that anyone of them ever exceeded the almost incredible powers of this modern Hercules!

It seems to be quite the prevailing fashion among all professional strong men and prominent physical culturists to boast of a weak and sickly childhood, from which they have finally developed into manly strength. But Mr. Unger is the exception to the rule, for in his childhood, boyhood, youth and manhood he has never been delicate or sickly. Probably that is one reason why, in his maturity, he has proven himself so much stronger by far than all of his competitors. For in these days of awakening public sentiment along the lines of physical improvement, when, indeed, almost every circus, vaudeville and even dime museum exhibits a "strong man" not one has been found who could duplicate or even approach the marvellous feats of Strength performed by this "Roi du Muscle," as Mr. Unger was named by the medical authorities and press of France.

Max Unger was born in Berlin, in 1878, of healthy German parents, but at an early age came to America with his father and mother. In his early youth he displayed evidence of a phenomenal strength, and gave his first public exhibition in 1897. From that date up until 1905 his time was divided between personal instruction in physical cult life and exhibitions of strength in the leading theatres of both Europe and America, though chiefly in England and the Continental countries.

At each and every performance he was accustomed to lifting to arms' length above the head, with one hand, a bar-bell weighted to three hundred and twelve pounds, a feat never equaled or even approached by any other athlete. There have been one or two wild and erratic newspaper reports of greater lifts of this kind, but they have never been verified. Even the far-famed Eugene Sandow lifted not more than two hundred and fifty-four pounds in this way, which is undeniably a very creditable performance, while the best other lift on record is one of two hundred and seventy three pounds, accomplished by the great Canadian giant, Louis Cyr. In connection with Mr. Unger's exhibitions there was a standing and widely advertised challenge to the world, together with an offer of a large amount of money, varying in different countries, to anyone who would duplicate this part of his act. Needless to say, aspiring athletes everywhere made the attempt, but in every instance failed utterly. Another popular feat was the lifting of a large basket bar-bell, containing two men, each weighing upward of one hundred and fifty pounds.

Mr. Unger is the only man who has ever accomplished the tearing of five packs of playing cards at one time, a thickness of two hundred and sixty cards. Sandow's best performance in this line was three packs. Another favorite "stunt" of Mr. Unger was the turning of a back somersault with a fifty-six-pound dumbbell in each hand.

But perhaps one of his most remarkable performances was his famous automobile act. In this he supported upon his chest, unaided, a bridge of about a thousand pounds' weight, over which was driven an automobile containing four to six men. In many cities autos of sixty horsepower were used, and in some instances electric cars, which are always exceedingly heavy, by reason of the great metallic storage batteries which they carry. In such cases the combined weight of bridge, automobile and passengers approximated eight thousand pounds. It should be noted that this feat depends upon the tremendous muscular strength of the performer. Indeed, Mr. Unger had some bones broken when he first attempted it, for the reason that he then thought of depending chiefly upon the strength of his bones, which, however, proved unequal to the strain. Later, when he learned to control and use his muscles properly for this feat, he accomplished it. He is also an accomplished boxer, wrestler, bicycle rider, and excels in other sports. He weighs 175 pounds.

A remarkable thing about this peerless athlete is the fact that his marvellous strength has not been acquired at the expense of health, vitality or long life, as seems to be the case with many professional "strong men", but conjointly with the very best of health. In spite of his hard training and the tremendous strain upon his system, entailed by his almost constant exhibition work, he is now in better condition than ever before, and is gaining in endurance, health and energy. This is partly because of his naturally powerful constitution, enabling him to endure the severe strain of such work, but partly also because he has always carefully and scientifically studied the fundamental principles of physical training and has avoided the many errors which others frequently fall into. He has always been temperate and careful in his habits, whereas the use of tobacco and alcohol, together with other forms of dissipation, arc fairly common among' wrestlers and so-called strong men. Mr. Unger is furthermore a vegetarian, having proven by actual experience with both kinds of diet that the vegetarian plan is infinitely superior to the practice of using meat in large quantities. This is another reason why his condition generally is so much better than that of his competitors, who invariably eat tremendous quantities of beef. In every way he lives a clean and wholesome life.

All over the world Mr. Unger has been pronounced by experts, artists and medical authorities to be the most perfect and most symmetrical man ever seen. At the request of the German Government, Prof. Louis Tuaillon, of Rome, Italy, made a statue in marble of Mr. Unger, which is now erected in the National Art Gallery at Berlin, Germany.

The famous European artist, Max Klinger, also considered Max Unger the ideal of symmetrical and athletic beauty, and found in him the inspiration to create several of his masterpieces.

Intelligence in Physical Culture

By MAX UNGER

The very title of this little book seems to imply that there is such a thing as physical culture without Intelligence, or rather, attempted physical culture, for without intelligent direction and a knowledge of the body and its needs the supposed training may be physical destruction rather than any true culture.

There are many who fancy that they need no special know ledge in order to been me strong and vigorous, but that if they merely exercise in sonic way or another the results will conic. It is true that such a course is often of benefit, but on the other hand, also, it is often detrimental. The novice, struggling blindly to get strong, is apt to make all manner of mistakes in his ignorance and when dealing with such a precious com-modity as vitality one cannot a fiord to experiment. The fact that there are thousands who have attempted some form of physical improvement without proper guidance, but who have signally failed to accomplish such improvement, is evidence of just as great a need for definite knowledge in connection with physical education as in connection with the development of the mind.

Work versus Exercise

Some there are who decry the practice of systematic physical culture, and recommend good, honest work as a satisfactory and sufficient means of building muscular tissue and promoting vigor. The toll} of this, however, is obvious even to those who have never given the subject any special study, for among the millions of the workers of the world there are extremely few who can claim anything like a symmetrical or athletic development. Nearly all forms of labor are such as to overwork certain parts of the body, while neglecting the muscles of other parts. But in addition to the one-sided development thus brought about, most forms of manual work are of a tedious and exhausting character: they consume but do not build strength: they drain one's vitality, bend his back, stiffen his joints and make him angular and slow. It is true that there are a few varieties of "honest toil" which might he physically beneficial to anyone, but the prevailing long hours for work more than offset the good results that might accrue in such cases, and the fact remains that most laborers are sadly lacking in any true bodily culture.

Women and Housework

In the case of women, especially, these remarks apply with great force, and in spite of the fact that general housework has been repeatedly, though mistakenly, recommended as a form of beneficial exercise. If only a limited amount of it is done, and that energetically it may be of some slight advantage, but the wrecked and shapeless figures of millions of housewives throughout the entire civilized world, after a number of years of domestic service, stand out as incontestable evidence that housework cannot take the place of systematic exercise. It not only fails to strengthen or to promote the health of a woman, but in most cases saps her strength and undermines her health.

Athletic Games Insufficient

Again there are those who fancy that athletic sports will take the place of rational, systematic training. The writer certainly should be the last to object to games and athletic sports of any kind; indeed, he practices and advocates them warmly. But in the majority of cases they are far from sufficient to answer all requirements in the way of uniform and symmetrical development or even of that strength and vigor which are necessary in the games themselves. An athletic pastime, like some special form of work, usually involves the use of certain muscles or sets of muscles at the expense of others, and the result is a one-sided development. Everyone who is familiar with athletes or athletics is also familiar with the fact that a large majority of them are far from symmetrical or well built, that they are round-shouldered more often than otherwise, sometimes flat-chested, frequently awkward and ungainly in movement, and that, when they are not too heavy below the waist and too light above, they are usually too light below and too heavy above. There are exceptions, it is true, but in a general way this disparity or unevenness of development may almost be said to be the rule among athletes. Notice it yourself, reader, the next time you have an opportunity to scrutinize a large number of them. As a usual thing, the so-called athlete specializes in some particular branch of sport, which accounts in part for his one-sided build. Strictly speaking, such a man is not an athlete at all, for he is incapable of anything but his specialty. The true athlete, first of all, should be perfectly built in every part, and therefore should be capable of creditable participation in any and all branches of athletics, including feats of actual strength, wrestling, boxing, running, jumping, weight throwing and all other popular pastimes. Special systematic exercises for all parts of the body are necessary to perfect the athlete, even for his best success in athletics, and it is a fact that the wisest and most successful athletes, when in training, depend largely upon the use of special movements for each individual part of the body, in addition to the practice of their athletic specialty. No one should attempt any strenuous, one-sided athletic effort until he has made himself fit by specially training of the entire body.

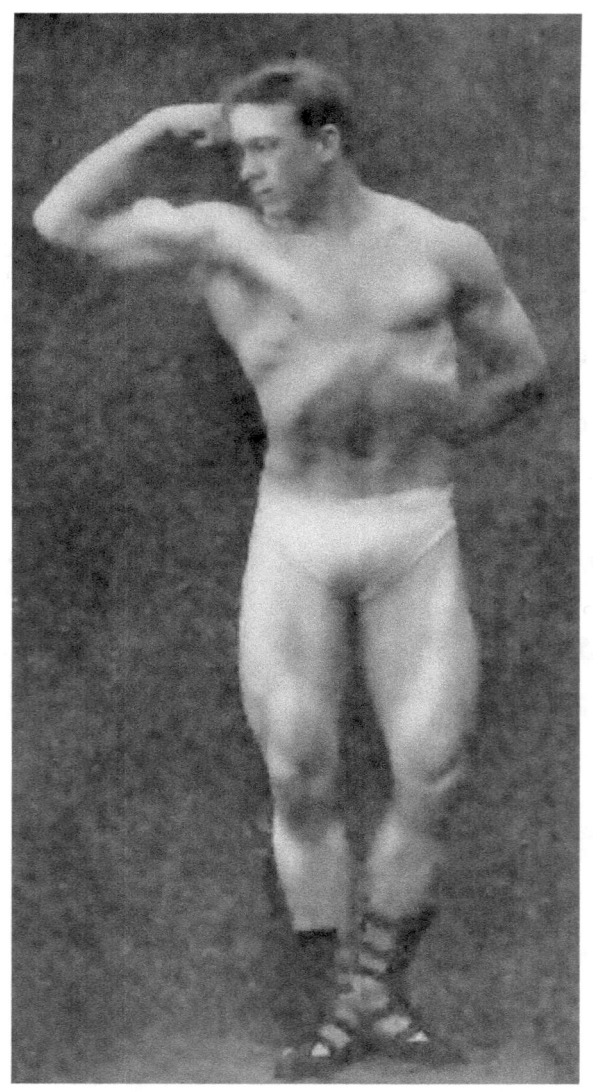

Symmetrical Development

But if mere games are not sufficient for full and complete development, the same must be said of many forms of physical training actually designed for all-around development. Thousands of physical culturists may be found who have depended, not upon athletics, but upon regular exercise, who are yet far from symmetrical.

Some of the most round-shouldered young men that 1 have ever seen have been among those trained for some years on the usual gymnasium apparatus, including horizontal and parallel bars, flying rings, ladders, vaulting horses and the rest. It is true that such apparatus offers one advantage, that of stimulating interest in the work, but this frequently carries with it the disadvantage of stimulating exercise of some parts of the body at the expense of other muscles. The "gym" enthusiast, for instance, sometimes develops a splendid set of arms and shoulders, to the neglect of his legs and the lower part of the torso. One who buys a "grip" machine may in time instill into his fingers almost the strength of iron forceps, but he may be a comparative weakling in other respects. And outside of the gymnasium there are many other examples of disharmony in physique, ranging from the track athlete who is all legs to the wrestler who is all neck and arms. Many teachers of physical culture, in their advertisements, publish pictures showing only face and biceps, realizing their lack of development in other parts of the body.

Costly Experiment

Greatly to our regret it must be said that in many quarters, even the teaching of physical culture is still in a more or less experimental stage, which accounts in part for the frequency with which those seeking health and strength are disappointed with the results obtained, as, for instance, when a neurasthenic has tried a dozen different physical culture instructors in as many years, without improvement. One professional "strong man" recently said in print that he "could not tell anyone else how to get strong; that each one must work out his own salvation" - an utterly absurd statement, but showing that he himself knew absolutely nothing about the processes of physical development, But aside from those who presume to teach in utter ignorance of the science and sense of health and body building, there are many others who are undoubtedly honest in their opinions that they have commendable "systems" to teach, but who really do not comprehend the requirements of the body in this respect, and do not take into consideration the many factors that are essential in an ideal scheme of physical culture.

"Unnatural" Systems of Training

For instance, one of the first requirements of any rational method is that it should be thoroughly natural, or in other words, in harmony with the structure and normal usage of the different parts of the body. But in many cases the most unnatural measures and devices are prescribed for bringing about results. In some instances, also, the development is "forced" along by measures which are ever and ever a little beyond the powers of the body to respond to readily. Such forcing methods are unnatural, it would be far more to the pupil's advantage and welfare if he were allowed to progress more slowly, but in a more natural way. Indeed, the ultimate result would be a greater degree of strength as a result of the more moderate and more natural development. Nature must be considered in these as in other matters, for no man can disregard or violate her laws without paying the penalty.

Complete versus Incomplete Movements

A serious fault with some devices and forms of exercise is that they do not afford "complete" movements, or, in other words, movements which bring a muscle into play throughout the full reach in which it is capable of acting.

The same objection applies to many games, which, despite their undoubted value, are not ample for all of the physiological requirements of exercise. Only by such "complete" movements may the muscles be kept pliable and elastic, or even as uniformly strong as they should be. It may be interesting to note that the chief necessity for special forms of exercise is due to the fact that in the daily affairs and activities of life the most of our movements are of the "incomplete" character, even such muscles as are called into action from time to time being employed in short, jerky, limited movements, involving only a small segment of the arc through which the affected member may be carried in a complete movement. When one's exercise, like the ordinary affairs of life, has to do only with movements of this character, a more or less muscle-bound condition is usually the result. It is essential, therefore, that one's exercise should not only afford him plenty of action, but the maximum of action for each and every part.

Lifting Machines

For this reason, among others, various patented lifting machines are very, very far from being adapted for general use, whatever may be their occasional value, likewise doubtful, as a means of testing strength. Even if the resistance offered were of a satisfactory character, the limited sphere of action, often extending over not more than two or three inches, sometimes even less, would condemn them. Like incomplete movements of all types, they render the muscles incapable of action except through this very narrow limit, and there is nothing more conducive to a muscle-bound condition, or to the general stiffening of the entire body. If one desires a weight-lifting resistance, it is infinitely better to use an actual detached weight, in which case the resistance will be found constant and uniform at all positions and extensions of the muscles. Perhaps one man in a thousand may find some expedient use for a lifting machine but for the ordinary man, who only wishes to get strong, such a device is worse than useless. It can not even serve as a true tester of strength, because of its limited action. The effort required in its use is great enough, and may assuredly accelerate the heart action, but the effort is frequently too great, and especially for those of weak constitutions and weak hearts.

Tensing and Vibratory Systems

Very similar objections apply to a number of systems of so-called exercise without apparatus, classified generally under the heads of tensing and vibratory exercises. Some of the vendors of these exercise lessons make extravagant claims for their systems upon alleged psychological grounds, claiming to have discovered some weird and mysterious connection between mind and muscle which had never been understood before, and which will enable one to gain far greater strength than by the use of any other method of exercise,—just as if will power or mental determination may not be brought into play to an equal or greater extent by any other system.

The above objections to incomplete movements apply with special force to the vibratory exercises and most of the tensing movements. They also have the muscle-binding and stiffening tendencies, and while they undeniably harden the muscles, it is doubtful if any great amount of real, serviceable strength may be acquired in this way. The muscles are not developed naturally. The essence of such exercise is the resistance of one muscle or set of muscles against another, the entire limb or other member thus being made tense and rigid. So that instead of the various muscles of the body being brought individually under control, and trained to act harmoniously with each other, they are simply trained to antagonize each other.

The possibilities for mental concentration, furthermore, when desirable, are all in favor of other more natural systems of exercise. For the boasted use of "will-power" in connection with the tensing movements can avail nothing, because in the very nature of the exercise, the effort (or mental effort, if you prefer), can never be concentrated upon one single muscle, but must be divided between that muscle and the other muscle which is required to furnish resistance.

The claim frequently made in connection with these tensing or "antagonistic" exercises to the effect that while they offer as much resistance as the use of heavy weights, yet they do not strain the heart in the same way, is sheer nonsense on the face of it. To secure the same resistance with the antagonistic exercises, the strain upon the heart must be and is just twice as great, for there is double the effort and twice as many muscles are used in the same exercise. Of the two methods, the actual use of heavy weights is the more natural, the more effective and the safer.

Heavy Weight Lifting

The practice of heavy weight lifting, however, is not to be recommended for the average man in search of health and strength, even though little else is employed by many having the audacity to call themselves teachers of physical culture. The fact that they mitigate the enormity of the evil by the claim of a progressive system of weight lifting does not alter the tact that their methods are and must be detrimental to those not yet prepared for such efforts. Invariable the ambitious pupil is forced, from the very beginning, to exert himself to the utmost limit of his strength, if not beyond, the result being that he frequently loses energy instead of gaining it. Or, if he accumulates muscular tissue, it is usually at the expense of his nervous system and a loss of vitality. Weight lifting is not an exercise for those who desire to get strong, but only for those who are already very strong, in which case it may be employed to develop further strength.

Deep Breathing Nonsense

Another of the most irrational of all physical culture theories is that one can secure health and strength by mere deep breathing. Not only is there no advantage in the practice of forced breathing, it is commonly taught, but the practice is even a dangerous one, and likely to defeat the very object for which it is intended. The daily use of apparatus for testing the lung capacity is especially to be condemned, inasmuch as it stimulates the uninformed or misinformed health-seeker to extreme efforts in this unfortunate direction. It all reminds one of the fable about the bullfrog who wished to inflate himself to the size of a cow, who blew himself up, and blew, and blew and finally burst. As a museum freak one might be very proud to be able to blow up his chest to the dimensions of a hot-air balloon, but for the normal man the practice is absurd.

In the first place, forced breathing is not natural. Nature has provided for us adequately in this respect. All that one requires from the lungs is the thorough oxygenation of the blood, and this is fully accomplished by normal breathing, if the air is pure. There can, therefore, be no advantage in breathing twice as much air. The lungs are self-adjusting, operating automatically, and when a greater supply of oxygen is required, as during vigorous exercise, the breathing is accelerated lo answer to the demand, Voluntary deep breathing when not engaged in exercise will not add to one's energy in the least, nor make his health more perfect.

On the contrary, the danger of such a practice is so serious that every one should be warned of it. An excessive development of lung cells is a far worse condition than an insufficient development, for the latter will be easily overcome by natural living. Forced breathing is not such all interesting or fascinating practice that it is likely to be kept up all one's life. The enthusiast may follow it for a year or two, and then gradually neglect it, with the result that he has developed a large area of lung cells which he no longer uses, which in his future life-time he will never use, and which, unused, will gradually disintegrate and develop disease, offering a fertile soil for the ravages of the tubercle bacilli. Athletes who have died of consumption have sometimes been said to have done so because of weak lungs, but in most such cases it has been because of excessive lung development acquired some time previous, these lung cells being later unused and degenerating in the manner mentioned. It is a danger that no one can afford to ignore. The large mortality from consumption among glass blowers is due not so much to the inhalation of dust, as commonly supposed, as to the fact that they over develop their lungs in their work. A period of unemployment will then almost surely bring on the disease.

Let one take a proper amount of active exercise for his muscles and he will need no special attention to his breathing. It is desirable that one's chest be round and full, giving plenty of room for the heart and lungs, but suitable exercise will bring this about, and brisk walking, running, boxing, wrestling or general bodily exercise will induce all the breathing that is good for one. It is only necessary to make sure that the air is fresh and pure. And in regard to the much exploited diaphragmatic breathing, it may be said briefly that every one breathes that way instinctively and naturally - every one except the tightly corseted woman, and she is hopeless anyway. It is not necessary to learn it from high priced instructors.

Delusion about Health without Strength

Another very common error is the delusion that health is possible without strength. It is true that in its best sense physical culture means more than mere muscle building, but it is also true that strength is an absolute essential in securing and maintaining any degree of health which is worthy of the name.

There are those who, themselves lacking in muscular vigor, are prone to speak contemptuously of the same, declaring that what they desire is not great, "ugly" muscles, but just health! It occasionally happens also that some weakling, verily "a rag, a bone and a hank of hair", will declare that he is in perfect health, inasmuch as he is out of bed and able to walk around a bit.

But as a matter of fact, no one can enjoy a high degree of health unless he represents a high standard of physical vigor. He should be a good specimen of animal life. And this means that he must be at least normally strong. What would we think of the health of a horse or dog that was not thoroughly alive with active, energetic muscles? Normally, muscle makes up nearly one-half of the bulk of the human body, or almost three times as much as any other tissue or system. The greater part of our food is consumed in the muscles, and two-thirds o£ our vital heat is produced by them. For good health, therefore, it is important that the bulk of muscle should constitute at least forty-three per cent of that of the entire body, and that this tissue should be in the very best condition. A good circulation absolutely depends upon sufficient active exercise for these muscles, as does also the proper action of all the vital and functional organs, which readily lose tone and vigor without the tonic effect of such exercise. In the human body, as throughout all Nature, activity is the law of life, whereas stagnation means decay and ultimate death. How absurd, therefore, the notion that physical frailty may be consistent with good health. It is not sufficient that one should eat carefully, enjoy pure air or even breathe deeply. One must be STRONG, with the stamina and strength of manhood, or with the vigor of robust womanhood.

You Are Not Too Old

Perhaps you are one of those who think that they are too old. If so, think it no longer. Physical activity should be continued to the very end. When one reaches the point at which such activity is utterly impossible, then truly, he is only a step from the end.

It is commonly supposed that weakening and stiffening of the body is the result of age, but it would be nearer the truth to say that age is the result of a weakening and stiffening of the muscles. Youth is a period of activity, and one can retain youth only by continuing such activity. Some of the most remarkable athletic feats, particularly feats of endurance, have been accomplished by so-called old men— old in years, but young in condition.

Perhaps exercise is even more important for men and women past forty or fifty years of age than for their sons and daughters, though the exercise should be of the right kind. The above considerations upon the subject of complete vs. incomplete movements apply with special force to those who have past the elastic years of youth. The many years of incomplete movements in the daily affairs of life have gradually limited the action possibilities of their muscles, and stiffened them as well, and in order to retain health and youth up to their declining days, it is especially necessary that they should take regular exercise of a kind to preserve elasticity as well as the strength of their muscles.

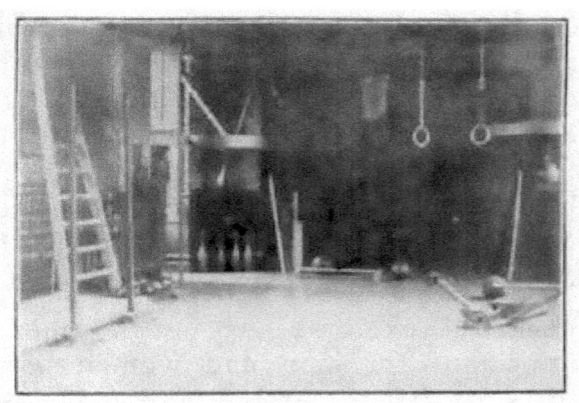

A Corner of the Gymnasium.

INSTRUCTION BY MAIL

Although I have given a part of my time for the past twelve years to instruction in health and body building, yet 1 have never before been situated in such a way that I could extend the circle of my work in this direction. At present 1 have a beautifully light and airy gymnasium on 125th Street, New York City, with which is combined the facilities of one of the finest and most extensive hath systems in the world. 1 have entirely given up my public exhibitions, intending in future to devote all of my energies to the work of improving human bodies, and at the repeated suggestion of friends and former pupils throughout both Europe and America I am now offering my services by mail, for the first time.

It is true that there is an advantage in securing personal instruction at my gymnasium, but yet one can accomplish the same results in his own home if only hr wilt follow my mailed instructions. I have arranged my method of instruction in such a way that I can give careful consideration to the varying needs of each individual case. As is well known, most correspondence schools and mail systems of physical instruction send out absolutely the same matter to each and every man who is enrolled as a pupil. Irrespective of the general merits of such instruction, when it has merit, it must inevitably prove an injustice to a large per cent age of patrons. In my courses of instruction, however, I supply special and distinct exercises for those of weak constitutions, and radically different movements for those who are fairly vigorous and who already possess a moderate degree of strength, in each case carefully considering all the peculiarities of the individual, and giving such additional advice as may be necessary.

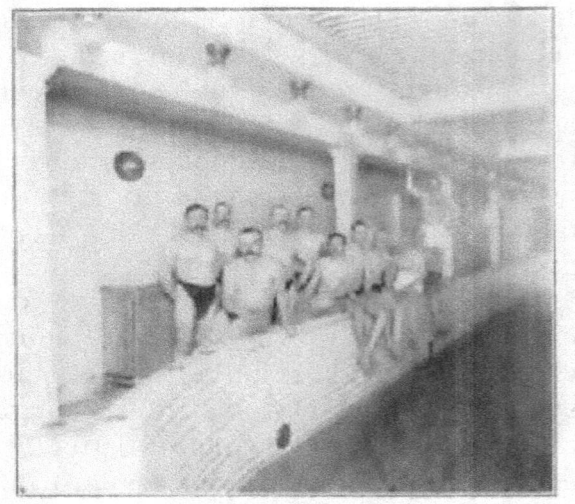

THE BEAUTIFUL SWIMMING "PLUNGE," WITH FRESH ARTESIAN WATER DAILY AT MAX UNGER'S HEALTH INSTITUTION.

Symmetry Insisted Upon

One great advantage of my system of training is the fact that I positively accomplish a symmetrical development of the entire body, a thing rarely known even among physical culturists. My method of accomplishing this is that of developing each muscle separately by the use of special individual exercises for each and every part of the body, no muscle or group of muscles being overlooked. Defective or weakened parts are given special attention, so that the body will become uniformly strong throughout.

The movements which I prescribe are of great value without apparatus of any kind, but in order to obtain, the very best results, and in order to secure a desired resistance, many of these movements arc performed with the aid of light dumbbells, varying in weight from two to five pounds, depending upon the strength and condition of each individual. Upon careful consideration of the question and measurement blank of each pupil, I determine just what weight of dumbbell is required in his or her case and then send a pair of such bells with the first lesson. They cost the pupil nothing, being supplied as a part of the course.

It is true that the dumbbell is an old-fashioned form of apparatus, but I have found, nevertheless, after years of study and experience, that they furnish the most satisfactory form of resistance for general purposes, and that better results can be accomplished with them, in the exercises which I prescribe, than through any other means. In the case of the elastic wall exerciser the resistance is continually varying, there being many times more resistance when the handles are milled far out from the wall than at the commencement of the movement. The same is true of wire spring exercisers, the resistance increasing rapidly with each additional inch of stretching. So-called "chest-weight" pulleys are far more satisfactory, supplying a more uniform resistance, but they are expensive, and like the wall elastic apparatus have the disadvantage of being adapted to only a limited number of movements, I have already mentioned objections to other apparatus, to which may be added the matter of expense. The resistance of the dumbbell, however, is constant at all points, being absolutely the same high above the head as one inch above the floor. And furthermore, owing to the constant nature of the forces of gravitation, there is a certain resistance to sidewise movements, and even to those which involve a quick, snappy pulling down of the weights from an elevated position.

The above applies chiefly in those who wish to become strong and vigorous.

For Amateur Strong Men

For those who are already normally strong, but who wish to acquire exceptional strength, perhaps to give exhibitions as "strong men," I can offer a special course of training, including the most careful and minute directions for weight lifting feats of all kinds. Please note that I do not offer this weight-lifting course indiscriminately, but only to those whose strength, measurements and general bodily condition are such as to assure me that they are physically fit to undertake such strenuous work. 1 realize that there are others who will teach weight lifting to any one, regardless of lack of strength or physical condition, but I positively refuse to do so. Where the applicant is not already exceptionally strong, I simply advise a general course of training. After he has secured a splendid degree of manly strength, I will then consider the possibility or advisability of his taking up the use of the heavy weights, if he still wishes to do so.

To secure the greatest possible strength, weight lifting is unquestionably the most effective method of development, provided the work is not forced too much, and a moderate, rational system of progression is employed. Weight lifting is far safer and in every way superior to so-called tensing or antagonistic exercises, and entails less strain upon the heart. It should he said that when one's muscles arc sufficiently strengthened and adapted to the effort, there is no greater strain upon the vital organs in lifting an accustomed weight than in any other natural action of an energetic kind. There is not as much strain as in the attempt upon the part a weakling to do some slight or trivial thing which may yet be beyond his frail powers. When the body is properly trained, even a great effort may be as natural and easy to accomplish as it is for a child to run or a kitten to play. At the same time, extreme measures and too much forcing must never be employed, and in many cases weight lifting must not be permitted at all.

I do not guarantee to triple your strength in sixty days, and particularly if you are already quite strong. Beware of such offers. I do not guarantee to give you a physique equal to my own. I will do the very utmost with the frame and natural possibilities with which you have been endowed. In some cases I have increased a pupil's strength six-fold and even ten-fold in sixty days, depending upon his condition. The forced development may not he lasting, and if one has in the beginning so much strength that he can endure the strain of forcing methods of weight lifting, employed by many alleged teachers, then his strength is already such that it cannot be doubled or tripled except by very long training. It is better to build more slowly, but to build well. Furthermore, rapid and exceptional development, even in the few cases where it can be accomplished by forcing measures, is usually affected at the expense of some neglected parts. In my courses of training, I insist upon a uniform and symmetrical strengthening of the entire body above everything else. The body is no stronger than its weakest part, and I see to it that there are no weak parts.

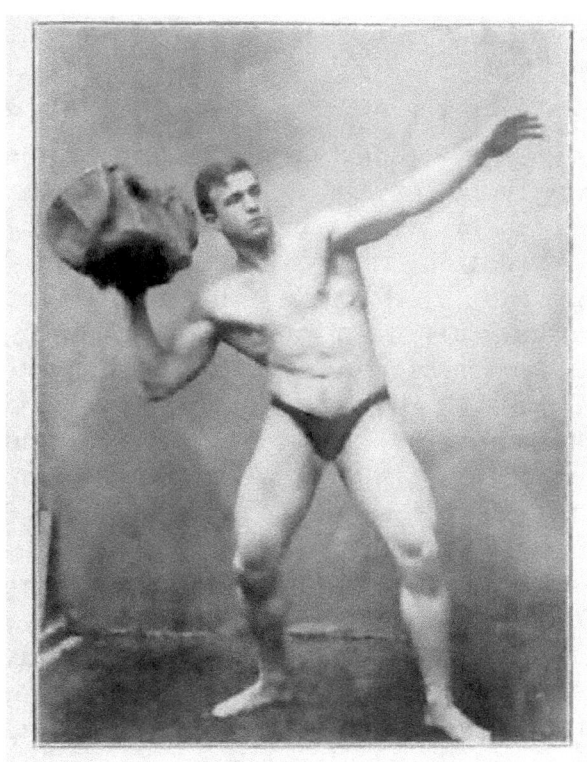

A Word to Women

It should perhaps be said that in my
endeavors for the improvement of
frail humanity I have not overlooked
the needs of our fair sisters, for
robust health is no less important to
them than to their brothers. Indeed,
of the two sexes, women suffer far

more from the lack of strength and health.

To be brief, I can only say that I am especially glad to enroll women upon my list of pupils. I have a great many of them who receive my personal instruction at my institution, and I give them the very best care and attention in my mail instruction, always prescribing exercises suited to their strength and condition. It should he known that, practically without exception, the weaknesses and miseries of women can be eradicated by special curative exercises, strengthening the back and improving the bodily carriage. Not merely are the muscles of the entire body developed, but all of the other tissues, and systems, organs and ligaments, are strengthened in such a way as to make pain and physical discomfort a thing unknown.

Are You Fat?

If you are burdened with superfluous flesh, I can help you to lose your burden. Obesity has its causes, like everything else and these causes are found chiefly in the lack of physical activity and in dietetic errors. There is no such thing as a man being unable to reduce his weight, no matter what his belief about it being "constitutional" or "temperamental" in his case. If only he will adopt proper measures, he can reduce flesh until he is down to a normal, natural weight - a point at which his health and efficiency will be the very greatest possible for him. I do not know such a thing as failure, even in the most obstinate cases of this kind.

Are You Too Thin?

If on the other band you have not flesh enough, I can build you up and enable you to fill out your clothes. Emaciation in many eases is due to digestive difficulties or failings, but perhaps more frequently is due to the lack of general bodily vigor and functional tone which follow persistent neglect of exercise, coupled with a conspicuous lack of muscular development. The individual is all "run down". But whether too fat or too thin, I can bring you back to the normal, to your best weight and the best of health.

Constipation, etc.

Constipation and digestive weaknesses, no matter in how chronic a form, can be readily overcome in my methods, which include exercises and rational dietetics. Drugs and physics only make matters worse. The body etc. must be considered as a whole, rather than as an aggregation of distinct parts, and constitutional improvement of the entire body will benefit each and every part. For this reason, practically all diseases may be speedily eradicated from the system by merely building up the general health. In this way, brain fag, sleeplessness, torpid liver, weak heart, weak lungs, rheumatism, general debility, nervous debility, sexual debility, irritability, impaired memory, kidney troubles, skin diseases, catarrhal troubles, weak eyes and practically all of the other "ills that flesh is heir to" may be readily shaken off. Merely give nature a chance. Gain vitality and build up the body, and disease will take its departure.

Vital and Functional Strength

I can give you not only external muscular strength, but internal strength as well, or in other words, that vigor of the vital and functional organs, which makes for untiring working efficiency, and which is essential to any real health or success in life. For it is, finally, through the blood-making and blood-purifying organs, that the body derives its energy, though as indicated above, they depend in turn upon the proper activity of the other parts of the whole body-machine. I have special exercises for strengthening and energizing these internal organs, digestive and other, just as I have special movements for strengthening the back and invigorating the spine for the sake of building nervous energy.

Morphine Habit, Alcoholism, etc.

In very much the same way, alcoholism, tobacco and drug habits may be cured, this being, indeed, the only rational and effective means of overcoming such habits. It is only the weak and lowered condition of his body that impels a man to use a stimulant or a sedative. If he were strong, healthy etc., and normal in every respect, he would have no desire for cocaine or morphine, whiskey or wine. If one is a drug fiend, chronic drinker, or a victim of some other habit, then it is my business and my pleasure to make him strong and well and normal, so that he will have no further craving for the drug, the drink or the smoke.

Beautiful and Attractive Pictures

A valuable feature of my course of training is the fact that the movements are not illustrated with cheap little drawings, but with beautiful photographic prints of myself. I have personally posed for photographs showing in detail all the varieties of exercises which I may employ in various cases, the pictures being printed upon heavy coated paper so that they can all be hung up on the wall of your room for constant reference, serving both as a beautiful decoration and as an inspiration to work for the acquisition of manly strength and symmetry.

What I Offer To Give You

I will positively guarantee a gain in strength of which you may well be proud: in fact, I will give you the very highest degree of strength that could be considered normal for a person of your temperament and build. I will give you a development that will be symmetrical throughout, and furthermore such an improvement in health, vitality and nervous energy will probably surprise both yourself and your friends. As a matter of fact, I will give you a greater degree of strength than could be obtained by too rapid forcing methods, for such measures ultimately weaken the constitution and defeat their own purpose. I will give you personal attention and exercises intended for your own self. And furthermore, I will give you such additional advice and personal suggestions as may be necessary for an improvement in the general health. This advice should alone be worth many times the entire cost of the course, and is an advantage not to be overlooked.

In order that I may reach and benefit the greatest number possible. I have made the cost of my mail instructions so low as to be within the reach of every one. The charges for the complete course, therefore, will be only fifteen dollars, a price far below that at which one can secure any other course that is of any value at all. I am able to make this low rate for the reason that I have no elaborate or expensive apparatus to sell, though it should be remembered that this amount includes a pair of dumbbells suited to the needs of each individual. Money orders and drafts are acceptable.